THE
GOOD FIGHT

SKIE BENDER

THE
GOOD FIGHT

SKIE BENDER

BLACKSHEEP BOOKS

THE
GOOD FIGHT

SKIE BENDER

ISBN: 978-0-578-17524-9

Cover photograph and design by Kevin Jacobs
www.FirestarterGraphics.com

Book design by Debi Bodett
www.DebiBodett.com

Printed in the United States of America

First Edition
Published by Black Sheep Books
Olympia, Washington

This is a true story.
Some of the names have been changed
for the purpose of privacy.

For Cy

a great fighter

Be brave enough to puncture your own viscera and explore the flood of self.
- skie bender

Table of Contents

About the author

Books By Skie Bender

PART 1

Punching keeps me peaceful

PART 1 - Punching keeps me peaceful

ROUND 1 - hands and fists

I am a boxer. I have yet to fight in the competitive ring. I fight in my own ring. Boxing is a metaphor for living. All of us are fighting. We fight to overcome obstacles in our lives. We fight to survive. It's with what attitude we approach the fight that matters. Boxer's exemplify the ultimate in body-mind-spirit-strength. Boxer's are ready to pop back up when they get knocked down.

In my mind I've always been a boxer, but I didn't physically practice boxing until two years ago.

Why not sooner?

Early in life I was immersed in other practices. A boxing opportunity never presented itself to me. I can only speculate that if boxing had shown its poker face to me in my youth, I would have instantly gravitated to it.

The first half of my life was spent surfing the roaring ocean waves, creating explosive abstract art and playing loud music in a rock band. I no longer surf, but I do continue to create art and play music, just not at the same cathartic level as I did it in my youth. I've always been drawn to raw intense lone practices that explore and express the self. I identify with boxing because of its pure primal animal alert instinct. Just me, my hands and fists.

ROUND 2 - fight music

I am training for my first fight. I don't have a match-up yet, because it's hard to find a pinweight in the adult division, but in my search for a match-up I train as if I were already on a fight card. That way when it happens I am ready.

I train at BB's Boxing Gym, an intimate old gym located on the industrial side of town. BB's is wedged between an automotive repair shop and a tool factory. Inside the gym the air is humid and hot, and the music is hard and loud.

BB is a soft-spoken retired middleweight champion with a dry sense of humor and an infectious laugh. BB's buff Latino wife, Gina (when she's not working out) greets you at the front desk with her big tooth wide smile.

The moment I step foot in the door at BB's I'm assaulted by the stench of flesh toxins, dirty socks and hand wraps drenched in the sweet 'n' sour sweat of passion for the fight. I find great comfort in the stink that oozes from human bodies in training. The odor rapidly takes on the flavor of a home cooked meal.

We fighters breathe deep and hard as we run furiously fast on treadmills, power-pedal stationary bikes, and let out exaggerated grunts pushing through one more intense interval of skipping rope, jumping jacks, lunges, crunches, and squats.

Synchronized sounds of focused breath, the snap-smack against heavy bags, rapid-in-time-rhyme on speed bags and the gut-crunch-crack of hitting hard-toned human flesh. Sounds of punching, punching, punching, sounds of vision come into fruition -that is - the sounds of fighters focused on self mastery, on being the best we can be, and for a select few ultimately being the best in the world.

My heart races and my blood rushes through me like a stormy ocean as I stand at the edge of the boxing ring watching professional fighters dance around and pound down. I close my eyes and feel the spray of sweat as it flies off the fighters flesh and listen to the low staccato tension-building tempo rising of blow by blow throw by throw cacophonic combination bomb drop down, down, down to the final count down 3, 2, 1 the bell ding-dings as the internal euphoric state of being exudes through the skin and permeates around the gym like a high and mighty heaven bound cloud.

Now it's my turn.

Wrap my hands. Zig-zag around and around the long cloth wraps across my knuckles. I build up an extra thick layer of cloth over my two big knuckles, the knuckles that take the hit. Open my mouth and bite into my mouthguard. Pull on my red leather 16-ounce beat-up boxing gloves. The ritual. I am in love with the process of preparation for the fight. The ritual that gets me psyched.

I have twenty-minutes to warm-up before my sparring session. Look for a heavy bag in the line of fire of many heavy bags that other boxers are beating the crap out of. I find a heavy bag that is not being used. The heavy bag for the purpose of practice is a body bag or my living opponent. Though this fake dead weight opponent can't hit me back I visualize, fantasize, work my defense as if the bag could throw a blow and knock me down, so I slip-slip, duck-duck, guard my face, guard my body, move left, right, back, and forward, tap-tap, whack-whack, power smack attack. I focus on fluid form, but I also listen to the tempo of every single hit.

1. 2. 3.
Jab. Cross. Hook.
1. 2. 3. 4.
Cross. Hook. Cross. Hook.
1. 2. 1. 2.
Jab. Cross. Jab. Cross.

I play the electric bass so I relate the single note tone of each string being thumped to the one hit fist pound sound resonance on the heavy bag. The bass is an instrument rooted in notes. Every punch I throw is a note. The punch-notes become chords the chords become riffs and the riffs become songs. Fight music.

ROUND 3 - skills and styles

Three excellent boxing coaches teach at BB's. Right now I work with all three so I can learn a diverse set of skills and styles to prepare myself for the real ring.

Jonah

I identify with Jonah's compact torpedo-like body, rebellious rock 'n' roll attitude, and wild-card workouts.

Jonah and I train on Sunday mornings. Jonah, a big Bruce Lee proponent, often refers to the methodology behind Bruce's one-inch-punch. Bruce Lee, one of the best Martial Artists of all time, delivered an explosive jab just one-inch away from his opponents' face that knocked them flat on their backs.

The *one-inch-punch* is more about brain than brawn.

To breakdown Bruce Lee's lightning-fast one-inch-punch one must understand that boxing punches take root in the foot not the fist. The fist is the effect of the cause. The *one-inch-punch* is fixed firm in the toes. A shock wave shoots from the toes through the balls of the feet straight up the legs, twists through the hips, rockets up the core, pitches the puncher's shoulder and fires out through the fist like an arrow right smack on target.

Boxing is akin to archery. Both are very present practices. Bow-Arrow. Glove-Fist. Bulls-Eye. Knockout.

Jonah instructs me: *Chin down, eyes up, work the inside, pop the jab, liver shot, side ribs. Small movements. No need for big movements. Big movements waste energy. Conserve all the energy you can. Strength is nothing without stamina. Staying Power.*

Energy Efficiency.
Energy Efficiency.
Energy Efficiency.

The one-inch-punch is rooted in energy efficiency.

Keep your body relaxed. Keep your hands relaxed. Only clench a hard fist on impact. Tension wears you out and eventually knocks you out.

Relax.
Relax.
Relax.

Erika

Erika is known for her knockout right hook. She's a stone-faced heavyweight with a body like a Neanderthal, broad and tall. Her slick black hair pulls taut over her boulder brow and thick bands of eyeliner accentuate her deep-set olive eyes. Thai tattoos crawl down Erika's neck, branch at her shoulders, and continue circling down her arms like aging tree rings. Erika's coaching style is silent and direct. Erika lives in a fight state. She doesn't make small talk or joke around. Her face is frozen in the game – poker face. Just being in her sturdy presence makes me stronger.

We train on Tuesday nights. We begin with a demanding warm-up set of squats, crunches, lunges, burpies, inchworms and mountain climbers. Then Erika has me shadowbox gripping onto 3-lb weights in front of a full-length mirror so I can focus on my form.

Just as Jonah stresses punching power starts in the foot, Erika emphasizes punching rhythm comes from the hip.

The rhythm is the same for every punch. Feel the rhythm in your hips. The rhythm never changes, get in your fighter's stance and swing your hips, just let your arms snap out like whips. The only punch that can deviate from the rhythm is the jab. Your punches are a team and the jab is the team captain.

Next we work the focus mitts. The focus mitts are flat padded gloves. The trainer holds a mitt up and the boxer mirrors the trainer. When the trainer holds up the left hand the fighter throws a right punch.

The fighter should never let their eyes follow the trainer's mitts or the opponent's gloves this indefinitely ends up in the fighter getting clobbered. To remain centered the fighter must always focus on the opponent's heart.

Erika sets the timer for ten 3-minute rounds. She puts the mitts on and moves her hands rapidly; left mitt – I snap a jab, right mitt – I power a straight, left sideways mitt – I throw a hook, right downward mitt – I land a hard uppercut. Then we work combos that are broken down into 30-second speed switches of straights, crosses, hooks, uppercuts, upstairs, downstairs, and of course *the most important thing in boxing* – Defense.

Erika machine guns rapid random combinations and I react fast by ducking, slipping, bobbing and weaving. She aims a slew of fast hard rights at my nose and I quick-catch and go, she strikes on both sides of my head, with my gloves held high I protect myself by rolling my face left and right into her strikes. Erika sneaks in a few lofty body shots to test if I am in solid guard position, hands up high, elbows tucked tight inside to protect my vital organs.

Move in. Move out. Pivot. Just keep moving. A boxer must keep moving to minimize the chances of getting hit, a moving target is much harder to hit than a sitting one.

Boxing is an art. But boxing is a hurt art. A good coach immediately starts throwing punches at you, so you learn to protect – defend yourself – you learn fast when you get hit and it hurts.

Mario

Mario is a stocky Puerto Rican Salsa-dancing welterweight champion with a dreadlock-mop of hair that he wears clipped straight up in the air. We train on Friday afternoons. Everybody wants to train with Mario. He's a fighter that's earned his respect; Mario has more knockouts under his belt than anyone else at BB's Gym. I feel very fortunate to train with him.

Mario's coaching approach embodies both the fast and furious and slow-go mindfulness. The majority of training time is definitely spent on the fast and furious. We start the session with high-speed footwork and quick hit mitt drills. Mario doesn't want me thinking, just acting and reacting. Just fighting! Just *Go!*

Go!
Go!
Go!

Don't think, Don't worry about details, we'll fine-tune later, right now listen to the hit rhythm, dance it, be it.

We begin with a very rapid lateral footwork drill on a portable foldout floor ladder. Mario cranks up the Salsa music and dances around as I jump in, out, left, right, forward and backward in this crazy boxer's hopscotch game.

Fast feet fast hands!
Dance the Salsa!
Fast feet fast hands!
Dance the Salsa!

Mario hyper-hollers as I race in and out of the ladder rungs as fast as I can while throwing snappy punches.

I love training with Mario. When I train with him I'm absolutely absorbed in the moment of act-react-act-react as Mario rapid-runs me through the ladder drills directly into the smack-attack focus mitt drills.

Mario's training style focuses on just bang it out and eventually you will figure it out.

Go!
Go!
Go!

Everything is repetition.
Repetition is everything.

Go!
Go!
Go!

Mario is so incredibly fit with such super-human stamina that he's almost incapable of understanding people that have only average to good levels of fitness. Some could say that Mario pushes fresh fighters too hard, I view it as a great thing to have a coach that believes in you more than you believe in yourself.

Mario eventually brings it down to deliberate awareness. To counterbalance the pure fight action we work on repetitive slow motion skill drills. Mario is wise in that he understands that the body needs to warm up and get loose before the critical mind gets involved.

Mario doesn't spend too much time in the slow-mojo. Just enough time that the body and mind fit perfect like cog and gear in a well-oiled machine, fluid and seamless in effortless synchronicity.

Try Easy.
Try Easy.
Now -
Go!
Go!
Dance the Salsa!

PART 2

Internal scavenger hunt

PART 2 - Internal scavenger hunt

ROUND 4 - obstacles

Right in the height of training for my first fight I wake up in the middle of the night with excruciating pain from the base of the left side of my skull, down my neck, arm and into my hand. The pain was so severe that I couldn't move my left arm. I was diagnosed with Brachial Neuritis. Not good for boxing.

Brachial Neuritis is an autoimmune related inflammation of the brachial plexus – a network of nerves that runs from the base of the skull through the neck, arm and hand. Inflammation of these nerves causes a sudden onset of unbearable pain and loss of full arm function. In rare cases, partial or complete arm paralysis may result. For most people Brachial Neuritis is a temporary setback – pain, weakness and loss of mobility self resolve to complete or near complete function in three to eighteen months.

This of course came at a time when I was the strongest, fastest and best boxer I've been since I began my training. At a time when my body and mind were in such a groove, fit as lock and key, that my training and myself became one entity.

In these fleeting moments of omnipotent jubilation life has a sudden and cruel way of reminding us that what we knew one-second ago is now a different reality entirely.

After all my hard work building myself up, now I was slipping back down and it was out of my control, I was angry, but like all recovery and grieving processes I had to come to a place of acceptance.

Nebulous thoughts blurred my vision I hung in this humid agitated state like a cloud full of rain that needs to burst, but remains bloated with a belly of water or like a hermit crab in between shells I was frozen in a state of flux, neither here nor there. I felt raw and exposed as my search abruptly changed from finding someone to fight to finding a new home for my uncertain bones.

ROUND 5 - recovery

It's been six months and I am 70% recovered. I certainly don't have the punching power and pop that I used to, but I am back in the boxing ring re-finding rhythm, regaining strength, speed and stamina.

I'm distended with gratitude to be back at BB's Boxing Gym because for the first three months after my Brachial Neuritis diagnosis the pain and weakness were so acute I couldn't even consider boxing. I can't convey how wonderful it feels just to put my hands inside my boxing gloves, even though my16-oz gloves now feel like boulders on my fists, I am utterly beside myself to throw a hit.

Three-months of intensive physical therapy, massage and chiropractic care has greatly improved my mobility in certain arm functions, the pain has subsided substantially, but there are pertinent movements my arm still cannot do. I may never be able to throw a fast hard jab with my left arm again. My left arm is my jab arm. The jab arm is the smart arm. The jab arm is the lead arm that sets up all the other punches. The jab arm is a boxer's #1 weapon, in both offense and defense.

If boxers are the embodiment of mental strength here I am put to the test.

Mental strength is everything. Mental strength matters more than physical strength because we can instantaneously lose our physical strength due to an accident. We can just as easily lose our mental strength, but without the mind what is the body?

If we are fortunate enough to be born with a healthy body than our body is a huge part of our identity. When our body is in a temporary weakened state we go through an identity crisis of sort, if our body is permanently damaged then we have to recreate our identity.

When our body fails us what have we left but our mental prowess. There is a saying – *We are not our body* – I disagree. When we are alive we are our body. Unless we are born in a state of paralysis, most all of our confidence and attitude depends on how our body feels. If our body feels strong we are much more likely to be happy and calm. If our body feels sick we are much more likely to be sad and agitated. The saying – *We are not our body* – seems applicable only when we are in a permanent state of paralysis or transitioning towards death.

PART 3

Self-service and giving service

PART 3 - Self-service and giving service

ROUND 6 - hospice

When I'm not boxing, creating art, or working, I volunteer in hospice patient care.

Hospice patient volunteers fill a void between professional caregivers and family members. At its core hospice volunteers give end-of-life companionship by being a good listening peaceful presence or giving the patient's loved ones some respite.

Hospice volunteer work also includes reading books or playing cards with the patient, meal preparation, household chores, yard work, running errands, and driving the patient to doctor's appointments.

The same thing that draws me to boxing is what draws me to hospice - both are pure, raw, absolute immersion into present-moment truth.

Boxing is fighting to survive. Hospice is making peace with death.

ROUND 7 - jack

Jack is my current hospice patient. When I received Jack's file from the hospice volunteer coordinator it stated he is an 87-year old retired wildlife biologist that specialized in Grizzly bears. Jack is dying from heart disease coupled with Parkinson's disease. He lives alone in the country and needs companionship. I've spoken with him on the phone, but today is our first meeting.

Straight from the boxing gym I drive to Jack's house. It's a stormy spring day. At the gym I showered, dried off, and put on clean clothes, but my body still feels sweaty in the damp air.

Jack lives with his dog, cat, and bird way out in the country. On this hilly rainy road I swerve and weave past barren fields lined with hay feeders full of fresh bales, but the cows aren't eating, instead they take cover from the wind and rain beneath boisterous old oak tress. High up in the twisted branches a murder of black oil crows tuck their wings close into their bodies as the rain falls fast, hard, loud as war on my windshield. Swift as a shooting star, chunks of fist-size hail begin to drop from the sky, I slow down, pull roadside, shut down the engine, wait and exhilarate at natures strange gifts.

Fast as the day turns black as night, the night cracks open bright as a spotlight and illuminates the golden fields, which are now snow covered white from the lash of hail, and something I hadn't noticed before a big old barn appears sacred as a church floating on a cloud in heaven with halo rainbow so brilliant so blue so yellow so true so red so alive so dead.

I turn the key to ignite, the truck coughs, chokes and spits. I ignite again and again until finally the truck comes back to life. Driving now with raised brow enlightenment, my eyes freeze wide in trance as I reflect on the disorder, the order, the cacophony and the calm that is nature's eternal collaboration.

In this moment the cold sun flickers through apple and oak trees, which are wide-welcome arms of bright shining green. Then the open road narrows and darkens as I enter a tunnel of evergreens and a soft quiet enters me. I am chilled from the silent beauty.

Jack lives and dies inside this tunnel of trees. His rustic brown wood farmhouse with missing shingle pieces is right in the middle of this tube of desolation. Jack lives alone. Not a neighbor is site. Jack's son lives on some acreage 25-miles east, so he stops by early every morning en route to work and late in the evening after work otherwise it's just the hospice nurse, bath-aid, chaplain, social worker and house keeper that are Jack's end-of-life companions. Now I add myself to Jack's list of comrades.

I pull my truck up on the loose gravel-hail covered driveway. Jack's dog barks deep-from his chest. My boots crunch-crunch across the gravel-hail that leads to a big porch strewn with broken wooden chairs, mud-crusted boots, paint cans and ceramic pots, which contain dead plants. The paint on the front door is so aged that I don't even recognize the color. The door is slightly ajar. Jack peers out. Once I maneuver through the porch obstructions Jack opens the front door as far as his wheelchair allows. Smiling, bright gray-eyes, vulture-slumped in wheelchair, Jack gestures with vein-shaky knucklebone hands, *Come in, come in.*

Jack rolls his wheelchair back to let me in. I introduce myself, when I extend my hand to shake his, he reaches out in great effort to reciprocate, but both his hands are shaking uncontrollably. I gently touch his warm hands.

Jack's gunmetal eyes shine deep and rich with his life's experiences. Big band backdrop music distorts from a radio in another room. The old wood floor farmhouse is cold, smells of stale coffee, cat litter and dirty dog. Jack backs his wheelchair up and struggles to turn around. I ask if I can assist and he shakily waves me off.

While I wait for Jack to turn himself around I stare up on the wall at a large framed black and white photograph of a man and woman on their wedding day, I can only assume is Jack and his wife. Once Jack gets settled in the right direction I follow him deliberately down the creaking hallway into the kitchen.

On the kitchen table is a transistor radio with a broken antenna, which is the source of the crackling swing music. There is also a yellow bird in a cage on the table, a porcelain plate with a pile of Friskies dry cat food on it and a big mug of milky coffee. I don't see a cat, but I do smell a litter box. A fat black dog with big brown eyes peers through the slobber-streaked sliding glass door from the wet deck outside begging to come in.

Sit down, sit down, Jack motions towards a metal-framed chair with foam spitting out of the ripped red vinyl.

Jack pulls his wheelchair as close to the table as he can get. He reaches for his coffee mug that has a big brown bear painted on it. I reach over and hand it to him. With both hands around the mug he takes a very shaky sip spilling a bit on his dark blue sweat pants.

Bright-eyes, stiff-mouth, crooked spine, and sunken neck, Jack starts in with his life stories. He tells stories about his wife, different dog companions, and Grizzly bears. All the while Jack's slurring, raspy voice fades in and out of the transistor radio music. I discreetly slide my arm across the table to turn the radio down, but Jack misses nothing, *Turn the damn thing off!*

Of course, now that the radio is silenced the bird starts screaming some repetitive phrase that I can't make out.

Can't shhhhuut that one up, Jack dryly points at the bird.

My gaze goes forth and back from Jack to the bird to the dog with its big moist eyes vying to come inside. With trembling hands Jack takes another shaky sip of coffee.

What's the dog's name? I ask.

That's Charlie. Heee'ssss a gooood ol' boy. You like dogs? Jack looks into me, almost as if he's examining me. Only a person that understands dogs would understand the breadth of this seemingly simple question.

I Love Dogs. Can I let Charlie in?

Get him a coooookie. Charlie's reeeeal protective of me in this daaaaamn chair. Heeee won't bite cha'. Cookies are back theeeeere, Jack flails his right arm backwards.

A big box of Milk Bone brand dog biscuits are on the kitchen counter between a large pile of newspapers, magazines and unopened mail. As I reach out to grab the dog biscuits I almost trip over the cat litter box.

I ask Jack where the trash is so I can clean the litter box.

No, nooooo, the cleaning girl will do that. Let Chaaaaaarliee in and sit, sit down.

I don't mind cleaning it.

Sssssit. The girrrrrl will do it.

Where's the cat hide out?

Mini, she's under my bed. Miiiiiiinni won't come out until you're lonnnng gone.

I pull a large-size dog biscuit out of the box. As I walk towards the door to let Charlie in he starts barking at me. He's bluff barking because his tail has a happy wag, he isn't showing teeth and his pupils dilate with excitement not aggression.

Chaaaaaarlie's all show. Give him a cooookie.

I slide the door open a few inches, Charlie stops barking long enough for a quick sniff at the biscuit and myself. I slip the biscuit through the door, Charlie fast-snatches it and takes a few steps back. As he rapidly crunches slobbery bits are comically flying out the sides of his mouth. Charlie keeps his eyes on me the entire time. When he's finished he looks up at me for more.

Jack rolls his wheelchair over.

Charlie, Chaaaarlie you be a gooood boy. Jack points a trembling finger at him. Charlie obediently sits. Jack opens the door enough so Charlie can squeeze his big barrel shaped flabby body inside the kitchen. Charlie slips right past me and slides beneath Jack's wheelchair. As Jack rolls back to the kitchen table Charlie crawls on his belly beneath the wheelchair simultaneously feeling protected by and protecting Jack.

Jack starts back in right where he left off telling me a story about Grizzly bears on Kodiak Island. I ask if there's a difference between a Grizzly and Brown bear. He informs me Grizzly and Brown bears are the same species, but Brown bears on Kodiak Island are a distinct subspecies from those on the mainland because they are isolated both genetically and physically.

I've known Jack for an hour and I feel like I'm visiting a cherished old friend.

The bird is quiet now, but attentive. Charlie peaks out from beneath Jack's wheelchair watching my every move.

I ask Jack what specific studies he did with Grizzlies.

Evvverythinnng! Haaaabitat, what they ate, where they miiiiigrate. Claws – three inches loooonnng – catch fishhh, boy can they fight! I was a fighter in my army daaaays thought I was hot stuff until I saaaaw them beeeeaaars fight.

Fighter? My spine and ears prick up. What kind of fighter?

Boxing, best in my arrrrrmmmy weight class! Jack lifts his fists as high into the air as he can with a winning gesture.

I box! Emotive excitement explodes out my mouth.

Well, ya better watch yer'self. Weeeeaar head protection. In my day no one cared, no one wore protectshuuun. Doc' thinks that's how I got this daaaaamn Paaarkinsons diszzzease. Got whacked in the head toooo many times. My fight name was Midnight. They caaaaalled me Midnight.

Why Midnight?

Aaaaah, yoooouu have to wait til' next visit to find out! Jack glows with boyish-mischief grin.

Today I came prepared to assist a frail old man with heart and Parkinson's disease. What I wasn't prepared for was the honor. What an honor to enter into another beings life, a stranger's life, during their final days, hours or even final breath, to be present as a witness to this transitory state of being that each and every one of us will one day experience in our own fragile life. What higher learning greater lesson is there?

Jack died of heart failure just seven hours after I left him. He died at midnight with his dog Charlie by his side. Goodnight Midnight.

ROUND 8 - fearless

When we are true to ourselves when we show up for ourselves each and ever day when we go all the way - we are fearless.

When we are fearless we don't seek approval or recognition of others.

We trust our gut.

No matter what ups or downs we pass through we remain rock-solid.

No highs. No lows. Only being. Situations change. People change. We flow with change. Our hearts remain in rhythm. Look at a fruit tree. Rooted. Grounded. Leaves fall. Leaves grow. Flowers explode. Fruit follows. Sweetness is short-lived. But the tree remains rooted.

I have always had distaste for the artificial flavor value that people place on awards, trophies and praise from the press.
These trinkets of acknowledgement for achievements have their material place, but the temporary-transitory state of wellbeing that trophy trinkets give us quickly pass, and if we are not grounded can leave us feeling low after the high.

I've learned to always accept praise with grace, but remain neutral when receiving external recognition because it has nothing to do with internal peace.

To remain detached from the passing moment of external praise I'm cognizant of being the eternal humble student.

I've never focused on winning. I've always focused on learning and growing.

I grew up surfing the coast of Southern California. I spent every morning and evening in the surf learning about the moon, tides, swell, wind direction and weather patterns. Once I felt proficient in my surfing ability I began surfing in surf competitions. Though I competed against other surfers I only ever cared about competing against myself. I surfed in competitions up and down the California coast, Mexico, Hawaii and Australia. I won countless medals and trophies, which made me proud, but even at the time of receiving these awards I felt, no attachment. I realized the trophies were mere exterior icons more for the public to gawk at than the inherent true peace I felt from working hard at doing what I loved.

Due to life circumstances I moved away from the sea and into the city. In the city I started an art-rock band. We worked diligent writing songs, rehearsing, recording, playing live shows, touring the country and Japan, receiving airplay on college and independent radio stations, cultivating a cult following and were adorned with high accolades from the press.

What separated the other hardworking bands with talent that we shared stages and played alongside with that went on to become publicly successful-*famous* from my band that remained forever underground?

Friends. Lots and lots of *Friends*.

To our detriment no one in my band made time to socialize with friends. I use the word friends loosely because in the business of business as well as the business of art one must always be on high alert of who a true friend is compared with who wants something from you, a piece of you.

Every moment of my band's time was spent creating and playing music. When we played shows and the show was over we went home or back to the bus. No one in my band cared about the after party. The *friends*.

We had strangers come to our shows. Unlike friends, strangers are true fans. Strangers are true fans because friends know you and friends want something from you, but to touch a stranger's heart with your art, to communicate your truth with a complete stranger and that stranger finds within him or herself a revelation of their own truth, isn't that *really* what it is all about?

Luck and timing is a factor to being publicly successful, and of course being marketable to the mainstream is a huge plus, unfortunately my band never was in the right place at the right time, nor could we be put in any uniform genre box.

For twelve years we followed our hearts and expressed our unique vision. For twelve years we were a force to be reckoned with. Our strange abrasive, often times uncomfortable style of music was certainly not for everyone, but we did make everyone think.

Nothing stopped us. We stopped. After twelve years of incessant creating, recording and touring with minor public success, but major personal success, we band members found ourselves in transition, both in the band and in our personal lives. We all agreed it was time to take a break. In our hearts we had a sense that we would one day regroup, we haven't yet, and I feel our time has come to pass. What we had was rare chemistry - *magic.* Magic cannot be recreated. Magic happens once.

My band broke up before social media became a necessary vehicle to communicate with fans. My band played at a time where most *everything* was hands' on *physical* footwork, like boxing.

Though I still play music for wild joyful release my commitment to my boxing life has replaced my commitment to my music life.

In boxing I've found an avenue to release the physical, emotional, cacophonic build-up from life's daily mendacity, tensions and ridiculousness, from slow to fast, from hard to soft, from express to watch, boxing has shown me this analogous hyper-rhythm-groove that I experienced in being in a band where everything was amplified.

My need to be in the moment's internal-external whole being intensity is for me not optional but essential.

Both boxing and music are physical acts of spontaneous performance. Both boxing and music practices are rooted in skill, style, awareness and heart. On performance night both boxing and music boil down to one thing - being fearless.

PART 4

Ready, Set, Go!

PART 4 - Ready, Set Go!

ROUND 9 - pinweight

When I walk into BB's Gym for my training
lesson with Mario a group of fighters are
glued to the side of the ring watching Mario
in a wailing sparring session with someone.
That someone turns out to be Frank.

Frank is one of the most revered fighters
in the state. Not only because he's a great
fighter with a record of 41-fights, 35-wins, 26-
wins by KO (knock-outs), but Frank is a very
good man. Six years ago Frank lost his only
son to a battle with Leukemia. Frank now
volunteers once a week at the Children's
Hospital in the cancer ward. He also runs
a training camp, Frank's Fight Camp,
for competing amateur and professional
boxers. On Sundays he hosts a program for

underprivileged and troubled youth to train for free.

The bell dings signaling the end of the final round. Frank and Mario duck under the ropes, jump off the platform, down to the ground. The other fighters pat the guys on the backs and exclaim about this move and that.

Boxing gloves still laced over his hands, Mario grabs and gulps from an open bottle of blue colored B-vitamin recovery drink, which looks more like car coolant than a human refreshment. Wiping sweat from his brow with the back of his glove, Mario sees me and says, *let me take a quick shower and we'll get started.*

I nod intently and start warming up on a heavy bag.

No more than ten minutes later Mario ducks under the ropes, hops back in the ring, ready with his brown leather gloves back on.

Let's go! Mario shouts.

I hop up on the ring, slide between the ropes and before I even have a chance to upright myself Mario sets the timer and starts the clock.

Ding-Ding!

Mario never wastes any warm-up time because in a real boxing match there is no easing into it. You are into it!

Jab. Cross. Duck. Hook to the body. Hook to the head. Jab to the head. Slip. Duck. Parry a punch. Pivot. Power shot. Duck. Jab. Jab. Jab. Parry. Tap and go!

We work nonstop around the clock for five, three-minute rounds. On my thirty-second break Mario has me dropping to the floor to do ten push-ups. There is no break.

Frank is outside the ropes watching me.

When the workout is finished Frank shouts over to Mario, *Who is the powerful pin weight?*

Mario introduces me to Frank. Frank launches a fast right rocket handshake. His bright green eyes shine wide with his smile as he unknowingly crushes my hand with his enthusiasm.

Like Mario, Frank wastes no time. He asks, *What do you weigh?*

98-pounds.

Hey, a buddy of mine coaches a pinweight out of Seattle and they've been searching for a match-up. Have you ever had a real fight?

No.

You ready for one?

Yes! My heart skips beats.

Pinweight minimum is 101-pounds. You could pump iron and eat twice as much and we'll have a match-up. Pop over next Thursday at four o'clock. I'll train you for your fight debut. Frank hands me his card.

A surge of adrenaline rushes rampant through me. What just happened? I open my mouth to say thank you, but nothing comes out.

ROUND 10 - frank's fight camp

I drive the beautiful backcountry roads to Frank's Fight Camp. It's the first day of summer, the summer solstice, the longest light day of the year. The sky is bright and the sun is bloated with hope. A warm breeze blows through the trees. I focus on my breath and how it aligns me. Oxygen is energy. Watch my thoughts as if watching scenes change outside the car window. My mind, like a deck of cards shuffles through construct and abstract images. My heart, full of gratitude for the opportunity Frank has given me. Frank has given me validation that I am ready for my first fight.

Car windows open wide, the smell of cattle. I sip from my water bottle, swish it in my mouth, but can't swallow because the water interferes with my meditation breath. I spit a mouthful of water out the window and it blows back in my face. I burst into laughter. Everything is irony. All is metaphor. Inhale water like a fish. Exhale flames like a dragon. My central nervous system ignites, but I've trained my body to remain relaxed. My bones, muscles and blood surrender to gravity as it pulls me through the car seat cushion to the metal frame of the car to the asphalt road to the fiery center of the earth. All is one and right with the world. I smile loud.

The road to Frank's is timeless. I drive through soft pastry pastures, buttery rolling hills, graceful horses, clumps of cattle, corn pecking hens, big gobble turkeys, darn donkeys, shy sheep, watchful llamas, squeal-joy pigs, slinking cats, barking dogs, and the occasional wild deer glimpsed browsing in the brush. Fresh picked vegetables at roadside farm stands, free range chicken eggs, country kids with lemonade, sugar cookies, picking berries, trampoline jumping, plastic pool plunging, oscillating sprinklers, grain trains, tractors, riding mowers, weed whackers, tree saw, axe crack, twisted branch, picket fence, big porch, rocking chair, fresh country air, everyone is outside working, playing, resting, soaking in the warm welcome summer sunshine.

At the fork in the road, go straight. Keep going until you fall off the edge of the dustbowl bison bath water wallow hole of the Great Depression Americana era of Woody Guthrie ye' ol' cowhand who never stopped roaming, rambling, recording and singing bout' the oil boom, dust depression and personal tragedies that swept hard and fast across *this land is your land, this land is my land, from California to the New York island, from the red wood forest to the Gulf Stream waters, this land was made for you and me.* You and me and Woody Guthrie, makes no difference that he's long been dead, for his timeless heart true songs sing on and on, and sudden as a car crash I begin to cry for you for me for the mystical mystery that is our breath.

I wipe my eyes. Suck in my gut. Straighten my back. Put on my poker face. It's been a vastly dry spring. Here on the first day of summer, seeds explode premature into large mutant fruits that on a Farmer's Almanac average wouldn't yield harvest for a good month from now. Haymakers start early this year. Hay bales scatter across dead prairie grass in whistling wind like lonesome tombstones await visits from long lost loved ones.

I begin my descent down the road into the tree groves. I am on the road to dying, not in an ill way, but in the way of enlightenment, I am infinitely cognizant of my living presence, I enjoy my life, I want to be with myself, not in an egocentric way, but in the humbling way of the universe.

Slow down, the road shifts from black asphalt to dirt and rocks, a raw road that parallels a pasture of cattle and crows. On this bumpy road I drive west towards the smooth hills where the sun will set, but not yet, now the sun is still so high and so am I, and so I am, in love with the fact that Frank's Fight Camp is hidden in this secret spot at the dead end of a dirt road inside a twisted tree grove, no one around but farmers and fighters, cows and crows masticating on fistfuls of fresh hay and a punch in the face.

Upon entering this enclave of swollen, knotted, hunched over arthritic trees that have gone weak at the knees is a discreet hand carved sign that simply reads: Franks.

My truck is swallowed by the dark mouth tree cavity, when I come out the other side the open sky light shines down on a rustic red boxing barn, with unblinking eyes, mouth agape and breath locked inside my chest I stare up at this big old barn as if it's a holy place of worship, and for me it is.

Parked in front of the heavy double barn doors is Frank's 1947 ½-ton aqua blue Ford pick-up truck with a personalized license plate that reads: HIT ME

I park a good ten feet away from Frank's pristine pick-up. I don't even want to entertain the possibility of accidentally hitting Frank's classic truck.

Before I get out of my truck I sit and listen to the warm whining breeze blow through the trees and it reminds me of Jack, how at the end of his life he lived isolated and hidden behind a wall of trees. I blink myself back from stone face memory to present moment, look up at the big boxing barn illuminated by the bright sunshine. Touch my boxing bag and make a mental inventory of what's inside. Boxing gloves, hand wraps, mouth guard, headgear, ear tape, boxing shoes, socks, shorts, protein bars and an energy drink. I feel strong. I feel ready. A bit raw from the past weeks workouts and my stomach twists with amplified nerves.

I step out of my truck into the bright sunlight. The sweet summer plum air relaxes me as I walk excitedly towards the big double barn doors. A large stone keeps one of the barn doors slightly ajar. I gently push the door open, a spear of sunlight shoots in like a laser beam and lands right in the center of the high-rise boxing ring. *Holy art thou,* my thespian celestial self whispers to my strong fighter self. The high-rise ring with the sun shining spot in the center is a ceremonious altar where the divine fight materializes. Just then, as if from the heavens, a voice billows from the darkness above.

Welcome!

I look up. Frank is hanging from a rope that's secured around a solid wood ceiling beam.

You're fifteen minutes early, which means you're on time. Frank says just before letting go of the rope and falling to a safety platform below. Without missing a beat he pops off the platform and gives me his notorious bone-crushing handshake.

Locker room that way, Frank points towards the back of the barn. *Gear up - fight ready!*

As I walk towards the locker room the solid concrete floor feels extra hard beneath my sore feet, bones and muscles from overworking my body, but I hold my head high and maintain a stride that's contained, like an injured wild animal I hide the pain. In the workout area the concrete is covered with thick black mats and the boxing ring floor is made from a shock absorbing foam covered by heavy canvas, so I won't feel as sore once I'm bouncing about in the ring.

The locker room has no lockers. It's a converted horse stall with open wooden shelves to store gym bags on. There are two long wooden benches for sitting. I toss my bag on one of the shelves and pull out my gear. Gather my hair into a ponytail, pin back any loose hairs that might fall into my eyes while I fight. Pull a small reel of white surgical tape out of a side pocket in my bag, which I wrap neatly around my ears. I have four piercings in each ear and the semi-permanent stainless steel earrings I wear are difficult put on and take off so I tape my ears with surgical tape to protect them. Otherwise my earrings can potentially get ripped out and make a bloody mess. I've seen it happen. Even when wearing headgear protection. One explosive hook to the head and earrings act like razor blades slicing right through the soft ear cartilage.

Sit down on one of the hard benches, remove my scuffed black street shoes, pull off my jean shorts, underneath I wear my pink form fitting fight shorts. Lace up smooth tread red boxing high tops, tighten and double knot the long white laces. With care I zig-zag long cloth wraps around my hands. Position my shiny candy apple colored headgear over my head, buckle the strap securely under my chin, wiggle the headgear back and forth to assure it's not going to slip while I'm launching punches.

Open my mouth and bite down on the charcoal child's size plastic molded mouthguard that protects my small teeth from getting knocked out of my head. My mouth fills with saliva. Boxers learn to 'spit-breathe' so we don't choke.

Lastly, I put on my right glove and tighten the Velcro strap as snug as I can get it. Then pull on my left glove, take the Velcro strap in my teeth and tighten it that way because

I can't use my hands since they're fisted up inside my gloves. Hop off the bench, jump up and down and throw a few punches into the air. Inhale and exhale through my nose, let's do this!

I walk slow and steady towards the ring where Frank is already gloved up and shadowboxing. I duck under the ropes. Without warning Frank just starts. He hits the timer. Ding! Not a word is spoken. We are in it. Frank throws a jab that I parry with my right and extend towards his face. He slips and counters. Frank's hands are fast. *Jab-Jab. Cross. Hook. Duck. Jab. Overhead. Cross. Shovel-hook. Liver-shot. Head-hook. Pivot in. Pivot out. Right-straight. Body block left.*

We work for a grueling action-packed eighteen minutes, which breaks down into three, five-minute rounds with a one-minute break in between rounds. Akin to Mario's training style (Frank was Mario's coach), a break does not equate rest; it means time to do push-ups, sit-ups and squats.

Ding-Ding!

After the eighteen minutes is over Frank points to a bundle of jump ropes hanging on a hook just outside the ring.

Quick sip of water then grab a rope and start skipping, he instructs.

Inevitably I am always forced to reveal the weakness in my left arm but I try and avoid it until it comes up. I don't like to start off talking about what I can't do; I keep my mouth shut and show what I can do. A disability in boxing no matter how small is a disadvantage.

When Frank offered to train me I didn't want to say anything that would factor in a negative, I didn't want the slightest identification with anything weak, I didn't want anything that would possibly jeopardize my chance to train with the best, so I can be my best.

I was so thrilled when Frank saw me spar with Mario and he seemingly didn't notice the loss of power in my left arm, or at least he didn't mention anything. I suppose this fact alone significantly boosted my confidence as a boxer. If Frank, one of the greats, didn't see anything wrong than I must be doing something right.

My hurt left arm has become my own personal test to see if I can pull the wool over every ones eyes, to see if I can still be top of my game with an arm that is partially lame. This is boxing after all two strong arms are more than half the game, but two strong legs, one strong heart and a hunger to fight comes into play in a big way.

At this point I don't see how my left arm is ever going to completely heal. I'm not being negative; it's a physiological fact due to explicit nerve damage, muscle atrophy and specific range of motion limitations that immobilize critical movements.

One such movement is skipping rope. My left arm almost bends into the L-shape needed for spinning the rope when I have no rope in hand, but once I start spinning the rope, my arm can't maintain the L-shape, meaning I am unable to spin the rope over my head. Skipping rope is an essential part of a boxer's toolbox because it's an easy albeit extremely effective method of attaining balance, coordination, strength and stamina.

I compensate for not being able to spin rope by just jumping. When I'm jumping along with other boxers that are spinning ropes I listen to the whir of their rope as it cuts through the air and the snap of their rope as it hits the mat. I align myself with the rope sound so I'm in rhythm with the other boxers as I jump-jump-jump with my invisible rope.

Hey, Coach. I say to Frank as I'm catching my breath.

Frank turns his head his sharp green eyes pierce into me.

I have to tell you about a small impairment I have in my left arm.

I wrap my left hand around the back left side of my neck.

I have this Brachial Neuritis, which causes nerve damage from my neck into my shoulder and down my left arm to my hand. I despise excuses, but it limits my range of motion and prevents me from doing certain exercises like jumping rope, it also weakens the speed and power of my jab.

As to not end on a downbeat, I chime in, *I can't jump rope, but I certainly can jump.* I start jumping.

Frank cracks a smile of amusement like a parent would give a child.

I keep jumping as Frank starts speaking. He tells me the first time he watched me fight with Mario he immediately saw my *problematic* arm. He and Mario actually discussed my injury, but Mario wasn't concerned, Mario told Frank that I've learned how to work around it.

Frank says that when we worked inside the ring today he observed my left arm and noticed a lot of drag on my offense and slow reaction time on my defense, so slow that in a real fight I'd be knocked out with a power shot to the left side of my head. Frank says he will show me some tricks to try and avoid that from happening. Of course defending the left side of my head will always be a very vulnerable spot for me to get caught in, but we'll do our best to have a smart plan.

Frank continues. *Quite honestly, the reason I was interested in training you is it's really hard to find a pinweight match-up in the adult arena. My buddy's been searching for a match with his pinweight for some time now. But that is definitely not the only reason, the first time I watched you spar with Mario I immediately saw a force to be reckoned with.*

Some guys and gals can fight, they are top-notch athletes with a lot of physical power, but sometimes that's a detriment because they just want to wail, and haven't taken the time to think about what they are doing, they haven't really found their voice, which is a boxer's style, what makes a fighter unique, and ultimately carries a fighter for the long haul. You know your voice.

One aspect of knowing your voice is it gives you the right attitude. The right attitude is the willingness to work through weakness and pain with a smile on your face. You have the right attitude. Your attitude guides you to make the right choices. One right choice you've already made is you don't let anything stop you no matter what the circumstance, that's because you know who you are and what you want - your voice!

Frank pauses.

Don't get me wrong, to be a great boxer you need great speed and physical power, but mental power is half the battle, with your fortitude you've won half the battle.

I listen wide-eyed, still spinning my imaginary rope, jump-jump-jump.

Frank continues.

I contacted my buddy and we're on the fight card for September 9th. We've got about ten weeks to get you more than ready. Here's the plan: Fight Camp lasts for eight weeks. We're just starting a new session. Camp is Monday through Saturday 4:30-11:30a.m. But you will only train with the camp fighters on Saturdays. You and I will do privates Monday through Friday from 5-8p.m. Good?

Yes Coach! I stop jumping.

Hey, who told you to stop jumping?

Yes Coach! I jump faster.

ROUND 11 - wild fire

Saturday morning. 4:00a.m. My first morning training with the other fighters at Frank's Fight Camp. At the early-edge hour between dreams and dawn the fighters arrive under a misty moon sky bundled in hooded sweatshirts. Outside the barn fighters shadow box at the moon. The dark air is filled with the scent of burning grass, cow dung and sweet plum. Fires burn through the hills, plains and valleys across the land. It's the driest summer on record. The rancher just beyond the tree line has already started moving cattle. Deep-throated *mooooo-mooooo* is faintly heard like a low note drawn out on a big cello.

4:15a.m. Frank arrives in bright white boxing shoes with a bounce in his step.

Morning! He smiles as he unlocks the barn door.

Some fighters' smile back, others just nod, but no one speaks.

Frank opens one of the two big barn doors, steps inside and turns on the electric lights. Lights flicker like twinkling stars as the fighters shuffle into the cold barn. Dawn's early silence makes it feel more like a monastery than a fight gym.

At 4:30 a.m. Frank hollers, *Line Up!*

In modern day warrior tradition the fighters line up on the black matt in front of Frank. In honor of the good fight, the pure fight, the honest fight, Frank places his hands together in prayer position and commands, Fight!

The fighters repeat, *Yes Coach!*

At first light we begin our fight with footwork across the mat. We work in a single file line with a lot of space in between fighters in this warrior wake-up dance.

For the person that knows nothing about boxing and assumes it's a violent blood sport of reckless punching, he or she would be quite surprised to learn that boxing is akin to a dance art form. Like any art form the only thing the spectator sees is the final product, in boxing that would be punching another person's face.

The conscious process of practicing boxing technique is not too much different from rehearsing dance in that both the boxer and the dancer must have complete body awareness. Within that awareness both boxer and dancer must be absolved in absolute moment-to-moment movement of isolating specific body parts. Both practices are deliberate immersion into aligning and balancing the body to utilize its full energy potential.

At Frank's Fight Camp our warm-up warrior fight dance entails the basics of boxing footwork, which in traditional boxer's stance is left foot in front. Move forward with the left foot first. Move back with the right foot first. Move right with the right foot first. Move left with the left foot first. If one is a southpaw, (right foot in front) than the dance is reversed. Most importantly, no matter which way a boxer is moving is that he or she must always remain grounded in fight stance.

After our legs are loose we bring punches into it. We step forward with our left foot and snap our left jab, then from the ball of our right foot we twist at the hip and throw a right cross. Whether throwing or blocking a punch the fighter's body twists into various angles so the fighter's core remains solid as a tree trunk to retain balance.

In our fight stance dance we awaken the sleepy dawn with our fiercely choreographed combat rhythm. Each time we throw a jab through the air we exhale *pssshhh-pssshhh*. Our heart rates rise with the smoky sun outside. How alive we become in this concentrated setting of full front sight fight focus. If ever our eyes wander Frank calls us out. Inside the fight ring a fighter must never take his or her eyes off their opponent. Fighters cannot afford to let anything distract them. Not paying attention for even a hairline of a second can result in being knocked out.

After fifteen minutes of footwork the wall timer beeps and Frank orders, *Animal Movements!*

Animal Movements are playful albeit difficult stretching, strength and cardiovascular conditioning movements on the mat. For a child the movements would be considered fun because a child's body is much more limber and bouncy then an adult's body. For adults the Animal Movements can be quite strenuous until practiced for a few months to build up strength and flexibility.

Fifteen minutes of Animal Movements:

Kangaroo - long leap and land, leap and land, nonstop across the 50-yard mat.

Stork - long leg high kick into the air than land in a deep lunge stretch.

Gorilla - straight-back squat position move quickly sideways as hands hit the mat.

Crab - backwards crawl with palms flat behind the back and buttocks inches from the mat.

Panther - push-up position, stay low to ground and bring left knee to left elbow and right knee to right elbow with stomach inches from the mat.

The wall timer beeps. Frank calls out, *Skip and Sprawl!*

The next fifteen minutes of skipping rope are broken by Frank's random shouts of, *sprawl!*

A sprawl is a martial arts term for a defensive block when one fighter attempts to throw another fighter to the ground. For the purpose of traditional boxing it is pertinent to practice the sprawl because it keeps the fighter fast on reflex in the event of a real boxing match where a fighter gets hit so hard he or she is knocked off their feet down to the ground. Practicing the sprawl helps the boxer be ready to pop right back up. The sprawl basically is dropping belly down to the ground with the legs sprawled out, and then immediately popping back up and resuming fight stance.

The smoky sun spreads across the sky and shines through the barn window landing on the black mat in a distorted rectangle sharp shape. The heat of day is in full play. The still hot atmosphere is broken by *whiiiirrr-whiiiirrr* of jump ropes as they slash through the air. The ropes spin round and round and slap-slap the ground. I jump rope-less up and down, up and down in repetitive punch drunk trance.

Break! Grab a small sip of water and I'll meet you outside, Frank instructs.

Outside a warm north breeze blows smoke from the raging fires in our direction. The glare from the bronze hazy sky makes my eyes water and my breathing labored. We have a five-minute break to re-hydrate and re-oxygenate so we can be strong for the next set of drills. I pace back and forth in effort to regain my breath. Unassumingly I look around to see if the other fighters are as winded as I am.

The fighters at camp train seven-hours a day six days a week, which is necessary to maintain such a supreme level of strength and stamina. Being in shape is one thing, but being in boxing shape is a whole other level, it's a much higher echelon of fitness than your average athlete. Even if you are a boxer and in outstanding boxing shape you will always find another boxer that is in even better boxing shape than you, so you are compelled to always work harder and constantly up the ante for yourself.

Run! Frank sets his stopwatch. Without realizing what is happening the other fighters' start flying past me.

Running is not my strength. Next to my compromised left arm, running is my weakness. I am always last. Partly due to my small stature and short legs, but mostly due to the fact I do not enjoy running. My entire life I have avoided running. Boxer's do roadwork so I can't avoid it if I want to be a great boxer.

Frank has us run through the tree tunnel ½ mile to the end of cow pasture and back. The thick smoke air makes me light-headed and sticks in my lungs. I feel like I'm inhaling butterscotch pudding. I struggle to keep up. By the time I make it back to the barn the other fighters are already gloved up and hitting heavy bags. Gasping I enter the barn. Frank, even with his back turned, notices how far behind I am on the run. Without turning his head Frank says, Where you been? I feel ashamed because I don't want Frank to second guess his decision to train me, and more so I don't ever want to second guess myself.

Excellent coaches have 360-degree universal vision, front-sight focus like a predator, very keen peripheral eyes on the side of the head like a prey animal, and eyes in the back of their head.

Brilliant boxers also see ubiquitously and use that information to quickly switch back and forth from predator (offense) to prey (defense) mode. Great boxers like chameleons are able to change instantly to confuse their opponent.

Physically intensive boxing training simultaneously trains the mind to be quiet so it doesn't interfere with what the body has to do. In boxing there is no time to think. There is only time to act.

When I am out of my mind and completely in my body, acting and reacting from pure animal instinct, when I am moving easy as essence, floating, flying and transpiring my human hermit crab cake shell of a body, when I am being and becoming a deeper higher entity than myself, growing internally in ageless ascension, even while my external skin starts to decay, than I am fully engaged in my love of life, in my fight to survive.

To grow is to live. To not grow is to die.

PART 5

Strange Circle

PART 5 - Strange Circle

ROUND 12 - special occasion

My hospice patient Joan is dying of lung cancer. She has been given three months to live.

Recently Joan moved from her home to a nursing facility. Once a week I pick Joan up and drive her around town to wherever she wants to go. We always start at the grocery store to get candy and crackers. Joan tells me though the food at the nursing facility isn't bad, they don't give you enough so she needs something in her room to munch on between meals.

Joan never married she has no family except for an estranged sister who lives overseas that she hasn't seen for years.

Joan is slender with sharp elbow bones that poke out of her thin skin like kite wings. She has enough strength to walk a short distance with a walker. When we do errands Joan wants to go in the stores with me, but if she gets too tired she'll wait inside the car. Joan tells me it's just good to be outside the nursing facility whether she gets out of the car or not, it's just nice to be in the day and watch people going about their lives.

Today Joan wants to go to the Goodwill store to buy a fancy dress.

I help lift Joan into my truck. Buckle her seatbelt and drive safely down the road. I notice that I drive much more cautiously when I'm responsible for another living being than I do when driving alone.

The humid morning air is stagnant oppressive gray, which is made worse when we enter the overstocked Goodwill store where a rank blanket of foul smells suffocates me. The thick stink of unknown human sweat hides secrets inside used clothes, battered boot leather reeks of rotting cowhide, pet dander dusts old sofas, and rancid grease from fried food sticks to kitchen pans. I humor myself with the irony that I find great comfort in the sweaty stench of a boxing gym, but today the Goodwill store odor finds me taking shallow-gag breaths. The difference between the stink of a boxing gym and the Goodwill store is I know where the smells in a boxing gym derive from, it's also easy to block out that bad part of something you love.

Relying on assistance from her walker and myself, Joan totters the short distance from the parking lot to inside the Goodwill store, but once inside she is noticeably winded. Leaning on her walker dressed in marine blue polyester pants and a pale yellow blouse Joan asks me something in a such a low soft spoken tone that I can't quite make out what she's saying. I ask her to please repeat the question. With her shock of white hair, fixed bullet eye stare, and smeared peach colored lipstick I lean towards Joan's mouth and strain to hear her faint whispery words.

Joan asks me where the wedding dresses are. She says she needs a wedding dress for her *special occasion*. I scan the store racks until I see the women's dresses then point in the direction we should head. I gently touch Joan's railroad track spine to give her bony body some support as she determinedly shuffles forward with her walker. Joan looks pale and exhausted by the time we make to the women's dress section. As she catches her breath I scan the racks for wedding dresses.

There are a few wedding dresses, I point.

Oh yes...for the special occasion.

Joan never says wedding. Never speaks of a boyfriend or anything remotely akin to a spouse-to-be, marriage or even attending a wedding ceremony. The only thing she repeats is *special occasion.*

I ask Joan if she's getting married.

Heaven's No, she responds.

I can only translate the *special occasion* to mean...death?

Among hospice patient volunteers we have a saying:

Meet the patient where they are.

Don't judge, assume, impose or interject any

of your own thoughts, feelings or beliefs, just be a peaceful presence.

ROUND 13 - watercolor

It's a hot hazy afternoon with an unsettling buzz in the air. When I arrive at the nursing facility to take Joan out her nurse informs me that Joan's health has rapidly declined, she is now bedridden.

I quietly enter Joan's room. She is asleep. I stand beside her bed and watch her fading face, listen to her labored breathing.

Joan senses my presence and opens her eyes.

She smiles softly.

I smile back.

No words are spoken for a few seconds.

Joan breaks the comfortable silence.

She says, *it's happening so fast, I didn't think it would be so fast. I don't have much time.*

I reach out and gently grasp her delicate cold hand.

She closes her eyes and smiles.

After a moment of silence Joan opens her eyes and tells me she has something to share, something she's never shown anyone, it's inside the closet. Joan asks me to open the closet and retrieve a box.

I open the narrow closet and pick an old wooden box off the floor. I set it on the table beside Joan's bed.

Open it and look inside, Joan whispers while making an effort to lift her hand and point at the box, but she is so weak her hand falls right back onto the bed.

Inside the box are a stack of watercolor paintings of birds and trees. They are beautiful whimsical honest compositions.

I've never shown anyone because they're not good enough.

Good enough? Says who? I ask.

My art teacher in 10th grade...I never took another art class, but I continued painting in secret.

It's art. Art is your own unique view of the world, your own individual expression. No one can judge what's inside you. One can judge illustrative skills, but these paintings are not technical drawings, they are color and design, they are fluid and beautiful. Besides, who cares what anyone thinks if it makes you happy, do it.

Joan's eyes get moist and wide.

I look away from her and back down to one of her watercolor paintings that I'm holding.

Joan begins to speak, I listen but my eyes remain fixed on the painting in my hands.

Yes, you are right, I would have had a much happier life if I believed in myself. Not just in painting, but in a lot of things. I wish I learned all this before I got old and sick, now at the end of my life I have a lot of regrets. I never made peace with myself in life, now all I can do is make peace with myself in death.

ROUND 14 - as the pendulum swings
Sparring synchronicity, tonight in the ring
Frank and I are one being. I don't miss a
hit. My reactive rhythm is as methodical and
melodical as the pendulum swings. I am
in a state of euphonious euphoria, feeling
loose free and in harmony with the smack
of my glove on impact, my bones moving,
muscles flexing, heart beating, pulse ticking,
blood circulating, breath inhaling, exhaling,
life giving, life sustaining tonight there is no
separation from within and without, tonight I
am absolute with the universe and myself. I
am not only ready for my fight debut; I am
hungry for it. I know these moments are rare
and far in between so I fly high. The fight
music is delicious.

Frank and I share this square ring framed
by ropes, not a sliver of a second is wasted.
Every second is lived. Boxing. Hospice.
Every second counts. Seconds left on the
clock.

Count down.
10
9
8
7
6
5
4
3
2
1
Game Over.

The bell ding-dings, signifying the end of the
final round.

I continue to fight, not as boxer, but as
not wanting to let go of this luscious bliss,
reluctantly I drip like honey down from this
great white puff cloud I am on, back to the
cold hard ground.

Regaining breath, Frank breaks it to me, he speaks clear and direct, but my ears hear his words as warbled chopping block sentences.

Pinweight fight. Cancelled. Postponed. Opponent. Broke her wrist. Recovery. Ten-weeks. At least. Reschedule. When. Healed.

A grave disappointment washes across my face like a flash flood.

I close my eyes. Clear and bright as a summer day I hear Frank say.

What really matters is not the fight that you are training for, but the fight that you are living for.

About the author

Skie Bender continues her boxing training, creating art, volunteering in hospice and animal service care and she works at Wolf Haven International, a nonprofit sanctuary for captive born wolves.

Books By Skie Bender

Riding My Big Wheel Too Fast
A Nice Storm For A New Birth
Collision With Fate
Indian Transvestite
Invisible Suicide
Orchestra Of Wings
The Knife Beneath My Shirt
Short Lived
Winter Sun